You're Not Dead Yet - So Stop Acting Like It! Copy

11 Tips From A Buddhist On Aging Vibrantly

Marc J. Sachnoff

Modern Wisdom Press

Copyright © 2024 by Marc J. Sachnoff

All rights reserved.

No portion of this book may be reproduced in any form without written permission from the publisher or author, except as permitted by U.S. copyright law.

Contents

Dedication	1
Introduction	2
1. Make Change Your Friend Nothing Is Constant But Change	7
2. Stay In The Present And Look To The Future Be In the Now	15
3. Shake It To Make it Make Health Your #1 Priority	23
4. Seize The Day Finish Any Unfinished Business	38
5. Spend Your Savings It's Your Money	49
6. Curious Minds Never Age	57
7. Snooze or Lose Sleep Like a Pro	64

8.	Write Your Memoirs -Throw A Pre-Memorial Party	72
9.	Simplify, Clear Out, And Release Let Go of Unnecessary Stuff	79
10.	One is the Loneliest Number Don't Go Solo	92
11.	Seek Beauty, Model Kindness, Accept Grace Live Vibrantly Now	102
12.	Afterword	112

Also by Marc J. Sachnoff	114
About the author	115

Dedication

This book is dedicated...

    To my father, Lowell Sachnoff, who modeled how to do well and do good.

To my mentor in life, the late Buddhist philosopher Daisaku Ikeda, whose accomplishments shine as an example of how much good one person can do in the world.

To my wife, Lynn, for her consistent love and support.

To my mother, Elaine Sachnoff, who passed away peacefully at age 92 during the editing of this book.

Introduction

Why Read This Book?

My uncle used to say, "Growing old stinks, but it's better than the alternative."

And Jonathan Swift, who wrote Gulliver's Travels, once wrote, "Every man desires to live long, but no man would be old."

Some think aging is an unstoppable biological force while others contend that you're only as old as you feel.

Either way, the truth is, if you're reading this, you're not dead yet!

Now that I'm in my 60s, I have found that some of my friends are living vibrantly while others are like the walking dead with one foot already in the grave.

As a long time practicing Buddhist, I have learned some key principles, some universal truths, and some really important advice that can help you and anyone you care about embrace aging with joy and grace.

First, a bit about me...

I was born in Brookline, Massachusetts in 1956. I grew up in Chicago and have lived most of my adult life in Los Angeles and Seattle. I spent over 20 years in the entertainment industry as a writer, director, producer, and development executive.

Then I got into the internet, the gaming industry, and ecommerce. Lots of interesting adventures!

I have been married for 36 years – to the same wonderful woman – and have two amazing, adult children.

2024 marks my 40th year practicing Buddhism in the Soka Gakkai Nichiren Buddhist community. As a volunteer leader, I spent much of my free time traveling and meeting fellow Buddhists across the West Coast. One of my goals was to engage with folks who had been practicing Buddhism for decades and encourage them.

Instead, they encouraged me!

These men and women had overcome so many obstacles and challenges in their lives: life threatening illnesses, loss of family members, poverty, language and culture barriers, as well as discrimination and prejudice. From these wise elders I learned many lessons about life, aging, living with illness, caring for loved ones, and manifesting compassion. I also learned about facing death.

At the same time, I studied the work of doctors, psychologists, gerontologists, and other experts on aging and its impact on our bodies, minds and spirits. Once I get interested in a topic, I'm like a dog with a bone – I just have to keep digging until I discover everything.

I have learned that there are some key elements, principles, and methods that can make all the difference between thriving and surviving, growing old and growing up, and ripening vs rotting!

I have distilled everything I learned down to 11 principles that you can use today to improve your life. Whether you are just hitting 60 or are well into your 90's, there's something for you in these pages.

Buddhists call the period from age 65 onwards the "Third Stage" of life. The stage is all yours. The script of your life may be mostly written, but the last act has yet to be determined. Much of that is up to you and the choices you make starting right now.

I don't know about you, but I resisted growing older. I told people that "60 is the new 50." I shied away from birthday celebrations and reunions. Then, at age 67, I was asked to become the Many Treasures leader for my Buddhist organization in Seattle. Many Treasures is the name of the group that was formed to support Buddhists ages 65 and up--the same ones who had so encouraged me in earlier years.

With this volunteer position came the inescapable fact that I too had become a Buddhist elder in our community.

Over time, I have come to embrace and celebrate my age. I want to share with you everything I've learned from my own journey and having worked with scores of other wise elders.

You're not dead yet! So you might as well start living vibrantly while you can.

These 11 principles have brought me and many others peace, joy, and grace. I hope they do the same for you.

Warmly,

Marc Sachnoff

Chapter 1
Make Change Your Friend
Nothing Is Constant But Change

Everything and everyone around us is changing all the time. This is an undeniable truth of life. Our bodies, our minds, our friends, our families, our environment – all are in constant motion.

Like a giant dance, the world keeps moving.

Our lives too are constantly changing. What is easy today may become more difficult tomorrow. While you might have been able to dance all night in your youth, a few whirls around the floor leave you breathless today. While not too long ago you could pull the engine out of that old pick-up truck by yourself, today it feels like an impossible challenge.

Changes in technology can be especially confusing and frustrating. Just when you've learned how to use your cell phone, they come out with a new version. When my dad was in his 90s, he was constantly calling my thirtysomething daughter to help him with email, web searching, and texting.

Some people curse these changes, railing to anyone who will listen, shaking their fists at the sky, and kicking that motorcycle they can no longer ride.

It won't help. It might allow you to blow off some steam in the moment, but take it from me, if you kick a Harley it will only hurt your foot!

It's natural as we grow older to seek comfort in what is familiar. We like things to stay the same. It's understandable to get upset when a favorite restaurant closes or a landmark building is torn down.

"Progress!" some will shout. But for many of us, it seems like the world we knew is slipping away and that can make us anxious and uncomfortable. It's as if a lighthouse we have used for decades to navigate to safe harbor has suddenly gone dark.

It's easy to get overwhelmed.

So if change is unavoidable, how do we make change our friend?

I've come to realize that while everything seems like it is in constant motion, there are some constants in our lives. These are not buildings or people, but rather something different entirely.

I'm talking about values and principles like love, faith, charity.

While intangible, the love we feel for others, the faith we have in a higher power, and the compassion we experience when we are helping others are very real. The joy that wells up when we hear children laugh and the fuzzy feeling when we hug someone we love are as real as any building or mountain.

Take a moment and think about the values or principles that have guided you throughout your life. What are those touchstones and how do they provide meaning to you now?

If you have trouble coming up with some of those touchstones, you might find that working with your breath is a simple and accessible way to feel grounded and comforted. I have also found that breathing is a way to connect with the part of us that is unchanging. Our essential self.

Anytime I start to feel overwhelmed or out of control, I know that's a sign from my body, mind and spirit to slow down. I close my eyes and take a couple of deep breaths.

There are many techniques for grounding and calming ourselves through breathing. I like the 7-4-8 method presented by Dr. Andrew Weil. I close my eyes and breathe in for a count of seven. I hold my breath for a count of four. And I exhale for a count of eight. I do this with one hand on my heart, and I match my counting to my heartbeat. Invariably, my heart rate will slow down after a few breaths.

Breathing to ground myself helps me get back on a firm foundation of faith, love, and compassion. I can picture the faces of people I love, favorite places or moments of joy from my life.

Sometimes, when things become too much for me, I've realized there are other things I can do in addition to focused breathing to calm myself and get centered. I can pet the dog. I can watch the sunset. You can do these or whatever brings you back to heart-centered joy and appreciation.

Then I can step back from the whirlwind around me and observe with a serene gaze. I realize that everyone and everything is energy – dancing and vibrating to their own tune.

It's not easy to embrace change in our lives. We might resist with all our might. Sometimes we don't realize a change is good for us until after we've fought against it and lost.

For instance, my mom swore that she would stay in her drafty, dilapidated, firetrap of a house until she died. "The only way I'm leaving here is feet first!" she declared, stomping for emphasis on the tattered carpet.

"OK," replied my sister (the strong one). "Then get your boots on because you're outta here!"

Up until moving day I still wasn't sure mom would leave. But leave she did. And we ended up finding her an apartment in one of Chicago's finest downtown residential buildings.

Today, she couldn't be happier. The building has a gym and a pool and a piano for her to play. She's in three book groups and a puzzle club. Now she barely remembers putting up such a fuss about leaving her house.

We might like to keep things the way they were. It's ok to curl up in a favorite chair and re-read a special book or watch a movie that still makes you laugh. It's fine to listen to that Steely Dan album whose lyrics you still don't quite understand or Beethoven or La Boheme.

Then I take a couple more deep breaths and step back outside into the world.

Paradoxically, my mom is also a great example of someone who embraces change. She loves hip-hop music, Korean TV dramas, and TikTok dances as well as the opera, the symphony, and impressionist art. Until recently, she traveled around the world teaching psychodrama, a form of therapy that involves role playing. And she was the oldest member of an improv comedy group, most of whose members were in their 20s and 30s.

Go mom, go!

The great Buddhist Teacher Nichiren said, "Blossoms turn into fruit, and brides become mothers-in-law." They say time is like a river – it waits for no one.

If you make change your friend, you will not be swept away by the shifting sands of time. Instead, you can be like a surfer who rides the waves of change, even as they roar and crash beneath them.

If you are willing to observe the areas in your life where you have resistance to change, you can begin to dance with them. Slowly, maybe hesitantly at first, if you can imagine a positive outcome from the change you are resisting, you will already have started to open up your life to new possibilities. You have begun to navigate change.

The people I know who are most resilient are those who have mastered the art of embracing change.

I once saw a picture of my dad after he turned 80 and realized that he now looked like my grandfather. But the real shock was the realization that if Pop looked like grandpa, I now looked like him! I had become my dad–at least in appearance. Fortunately, dad was pretty handsome, so I couldn't really complain.

The future is uncertain, but it's also full of possibilities. So be open to transformation, whether it's in technology, relationships, or personal growth. Make change your friend.

Journaling: Take a moment and write down two or three changes that are going on in your life today that you might be resisting. Then rate them from 1 -5 with 1 being "I'm not being very resistant" and five being "No way! Over my dead body!"

Now take a few deep breaths. You can close your eyes if you feel comfortable. I want you to imagine a potential positive outcome for each of the changes you wrote down. You can put your hand over your heart if that helps you become more centered. Then just let your mind go to a new place. Maybe there's a different way of looking at your situation, something that hadn't occurred to you before. If so, just make a note of it in your journal.

You can surf the waves of change. Or you can get sucked into the roiling tides. It's your choice. Change is going to happen either way so we might as well learn to embrace it the best we can.

Chapter 2
Stay In The Present And Look To The Future

Be In the Now

Now that you are starting to embrace change, I want to share with you one of the most important points of this book. This is a secret that will keep you young, fit, and attractive. Ok. I can't guarantee the last two, but for sure this tip will help you stay young.

As Bob Dylan famously sang, "I was so much older then, I'm younger than that now."

What is the real secret of staying young?

It's simple: stop dwelling on the past, stay in the present, and look to the future.

The late Buddhist philosopher, Daisaku Ikeda, wrote, "I hope that everyone can experience a third stage of life that is like a 'third youth.' Youth is not something that fades with age. Our attitude towards life is what makes us young. As long as we have a forward looking, positive attitude and spirit of challenge, we will gain depth as people and our lives will shine with a brilliance that is ours alone."

As we age, we have a tendency to begin shifting our gaze backwards in time. As our surroundings change and become less familiar, it's easy to seek comfort in the past.

We all know people who are focused on the past, or stuck on yesterday.

Think about the friends and classmates you had in high school. I'd bet at least one of them went on to accomplish something notable. Others had careers and raised families. Some volunteered in their community or served in the military. But I would guess there's at least one of your friends or classmates who didn't really blossom. They peaked in high school and flatlined from there, bumping along into middle and ultimately old age, still reliving the big game or the antics of the old gang. That's a classic example of being stuck in the past.

I remember a story a friend told me about his visit to a small mountain village in Italy. He entered the ancient church which was empty except for an elderly priest. Then he heard what he thought was crying coming from the back of the sanctuary. As his eyes adjusted to the dim light, he saw an elderly woman sobbing in a pew. Distraught, he asked the priest, "Is she ok?" The priest replied that she lost her husband. "When did that happen?" my friend asked. "Thirty years ago," replied the priest.

Sometimes it's hard to let go of the past.

I want to be clear, there's real value to memories. They serve many important functions: they keep us grounded in our history, family, and culture; they keep alive those who have passed on already; and they can be comforting in times of change or upheaval.

You should cherish the memories that shape your identity.

I also believe we can learn from the past. We can reflect on history, both our own personal history and that of our society. We can consider the lessons it offers, both successes and mistakes.

But I would submit to you that in many cases the past is like an anchor that prevents us from living in the moment and having hope, dreams, and goals for the future.

That's why I suggest the following mix. Call it Marc's Healthy Brain Time Allotment.

Mind Your Mind

I suggest you spend no more than 25% of your "mind time" thinking about the past.

I propose that you spend at least 50% of your time in the present. That means contemplating what's up for today, this weekend and the near term future. Who am I going to see, what do I need to accomplish? Who can I be of service to, and so on.

Living in the present also means to be fully present in the now. It means to appreciate the small moments: the taste of morning coffee, the warmth of sunlight, laughter shared with loved ones. Breathing and mindfulness practices can also help anchor you in the present.

Then I would spend at least 25% of your "mind time" on the future.

Wait, how can I spend time on the future when it hasn't arrived yet?

Ok, smart aleck, here's how you do that.

First off, do you have goals for this week? This month? This year?

I'm talking about goals for improving your health, managing your savings and investments, vacation or trip planning.

Are you making plans? Plans to contact or see friends and family. Plans to join or support a social or faith group? Are you starting a new jigsaw puzzle or a new book? Are you planning to learn or brush up on a foreign language?

All of these will help you begin to move your focus on the future.

It's never too late to dream big. Imagine the life you want to create. Set goals, make plans, and take steps toward them. Anticipate growth, change, and new experiences.

Someone once said, "One who eats the past is old. One who eats the present is middle aged, but one who eats the future is young."

You may not be able to accomplish all of your goals. Life has a tendency to throw us curve balls. As my friend liked to say, "If you want to see God laugh, show her your plan!"

But that doesn't mean we shouldn't make any plans. Absolutely not!

Make Plans

Daniel Burnham, the renowned architect and city planner, is often attributed with this famous quote: "Make no little plans. They have no magic to stir men's blood and probably themselves will not be realized. Make big plans; aim high in hope and work, remembering that a noble, logical diagram once recorded will never die, but long after we are gone will be a living thing, asserting itself with ever-growing insistency."

This is a powerful statement.

You might be wondering, "If I can't accomplish all my goals, why bother to make any at all?"

This is a question I asked a wise Buddhist elder when I was a newbie in my practice.

He responded, "If you aim for the stars and only hit the moon, you are still accomplishing something. But if you aim for the ground and hit your foot, you are just a moron."

I don't think the Buddha actually said that, but it was certainly memorable.

Our energy level, our mobility, our stamina, and our willpower all ebb and flow with age. So, we do have to set realistic expectations and priorities.

My friend Lee found herself single in her 60s. She was sad, depressed, and alone after a bitter divorce. To shake herself out of it she decided to set a big goal for herself. She realized that she loved to travel and always wanted an Airstream trailer. She decided she wanted to see the solar eclipse in Mexico.

She had never driven to Mexico from Washington – let alone towed a trailer – so she met a group of folks online who were caravaning down together.

Lee didn't know a single one of these people. They were all couples and she was the only single person. They mostly had different views on politics and Lee felt like a third wheel in a circle of fifth wheels!

But she is a Buddhist and not easily swayed. She was determined to have a memorable trip and treated everyone with kindness and consideration, even those who snubbed her. And guess what, kindness has a way of winning people over. By the time they set up their chairs for the total eclipse, she had made friends with most of the group.

Lee could have focused on her failed marriage, her bills, or her health issues. But instead of wallowing, she set a goal – an ambitious one for sure – and by accomplishing it she found new energy and revived her spirit. Now she has a whole new group of friends and has been invited to join their next adventures.

Go Lee!

Regardless of how much you may accomplish, I urge you to celebrate progress, any progress. Acknowledge how far you've come. Celebrate your achievements, no matter how small. Each step forward bridges the gap between past and future.

Remember, life is a tapestry woven from threads of past, present, and future. Honor each strand, and you'll find balance and stay young at heart.

Chapter 3
Shake It To Make it
Make Health Your #1 Priority

"My grandmother started walking five miles a day when she was sixty. She's ninety-seven now, and we don't know where the hell she is."

- Ellen DeGeneres

In the hustle and bustle of life, it's easy to overlook our most valuable asset: our health. We often prioritize work, family, and social commitments, relegating self-care to the back burner. But let me tell you this: neglecting your health is like driving a car without ever checking the oil or changing the tires. Sooner or later, it'll break down, leaving you stranded on the side of the road.

Here is a sobering fact: most of us will live longer than we will be healthy enough to enjoy. This is what some experts call our "Health Span," as opposed to our lifespan. Thanks to developments in medicine our lungs can keep on breathing, our heart can keep pumping, and our nervous system can keep our bodies going even though our quality of life may be less than we would really want.

That's one of the reasons that the last 10 years of our life have been called the "marginal decade." These last years can be rewarding and fulfilling or they can be a seemingly endless series of medical issues, deterioration, and emergencies.

I don't know about you, but I'd prefer to make it to the finish line in good enough shape to enjoy my final years. So, let's look at some simple and proactive ways to keep your body and mind in the best possible shape.

Dance Like Nobody's Watching

Remember those carefree childhood days when you'd spin around in circles until you were dizzy? Well, it turns out that dancing isn't just for kids—it's a fantastic way to stay active. Whether you're grooving to your favorite tunes, taking a Zumba class, joining a square dance group, or learning to jitterbug, dancing engages your body, mind, and spirit. It's also a way to get out into your community and meet new people. Plus, it's a joyful form of exercise that doesn't feel like work.

My wife is a professional dancer and I'm a semi-professional stumbler, but that doesn't prevent us from going dancing at least once or twice a month. I needed to improve my steps so we even took a dance lesson together. I still feel like a hippopotamus clomping around, but I really enjoy the music and the time together with my wife. I'm not out to impress anyone, just trying to have fun and not smash anyone's toes!

Walk the Talk

Walking is the unsung hero of physical activity. It doesn't require fancy equipment or a gym membership. All you need is a comfortable pair of shoes and a willingness to explore.

Take a stroll through your neighborhood, hike a scenic trail, or simply walk to the grocery store instead of driving. Walking not only keeps your joints limber but also clears your mind and boosts creativity.

Many people have been doing a program called the 10,000 Steps to keep in shape as they age. The 10,000 Steps exercise program has become widely recognized as a daily goal for physical activity.

The concept of walking 10,000 steps per day originated in Japan in 1965 when a pedometer manufacturer introduced a device called the "Manpo-kei" which translates to "10,000 steps meter." Interestingly, this catchy name was primarily a marketing tool rather than a scientifically validated recommendation.

Despite its marketing origins, the 10,000 steps goal has persisted and is now commonly used as a benchmark for daily physical activity.

There are so many health benefits to be gained from regular walking:

Cardiovascular benefits: Regular walking improves cardiorespiratory fitness, muscular strength, and body composition.

Mental health: Daily walking positively impacts your mood and overall mental health. Just getting outside and walking around the block is a great place to start. But the more you walk and the more regularly you do it, the more it can benefit you.

A study involving older women found the following:

- Sedentary women averaged 2,700 steps a day.

- Women who averaged 4,400 steps a day had a 41% reduction in mortality over those who didn't walk.

So we now know that you don't actually need to hit 10,000 steps per day to get the maximum benefit from walking. 7,500 steps (around 3.5 miles) is plenty and is a great goal to aim for.

Again, I am not a medical professional, and everyone's bodies are different, so before beginning any new exercise program it's always a good idea to check in with your medical team.

I have a friend who decided he wanted to walk the Pacific Crest Trail – a series of paths and trails that stretch all the way from Mexico to the Canadian border.

But at the time he could barely climb a set of stairs. Another friend said he'd go with him and they started training together. By "training" they meant two steps forward, one step bent over panting. Little by little, they built up their strength and stamina looping around a local park. Sure enough, they eventually walked the Pacific Crest Trail! Well, they did about two thirds of the trail... but hey, that's more than I've ever done.

Join others in stepping out. Most cities and towns have walking groups. You can find them on social sites like Meetup.com and Facebook. Community and senior centers also often organize walking groups. Or, you can just call a friend, a neighbor, or a family member and ask them to go for a walk with you. There's safety in numbers and it's more fun.

Embrace the Stairs

Elevators and escalators are convenient, but they can rob us of an opportunity to strengthen our legs and hearts. Next time you're faced with a choice, opt for the stairs if you can. Feel the burn in your calves and relish the sense of accomplishment as you ascend. Bonus points if you take two steps at a time—it's like a mini workout disguised as a daily routine.

As a friend once said to me, no one comes to the end of their life and thinks, "I wish I had taken more elevators."

I'm not saying you should run out and scale the Empire State Building, but when I check into a hotel or go to the library, I always take the stairs.

One caution, as always, start small. If you haven't been getting any cardio lately please don't over do it. Start one floor at a time and stop if you need to catch your breath. You can build up slowly and mark your progress.

Find Your Fitness Flavor

Walking is the easiest and most accessible exercise we can do. But more formalized exercise is the next step – pun intended.

Exercise isn't one-size-fits-all. Some people thrive in the weight room, while others prefer yoga or pilates. Experiment with different activities until you discover what lights your fire. Maybe it's swimming laps, cycling, or even kickboxing.

For many of us, as we age we may find ourselves losing muscle mass. Fitness experts say regular resistance workouts with free weights or weight machines can help stop the loss and even build new muscles.

Another common issue is decreased flexibility. This can be due to conditions like arthritis and a loss of elasticity in our muscles. But realizing that our muscles aren't as supple as they once were requires us to find new ways to keep fit and flexible. My favorite activity for flexibility, stamina, and balance is yoga. Whether you're sweating it out with 100 strangers in a hot yoga studio or sitting for chair yoga, I believe any yoga is better than no yoga.

But one word of caution: always consult your physician or medical team before starting a new exercise routine. Make sure you are starting slowly. Even riding a bike – although everyone says you never forget – requires re-acquainting yourself with balance, effort, and agility.

And don't feel like you have to compete with the 20 or 30 somethings in the front of the class. I once tried keeping up with the kid in front of me in a stationary bike spinning class and ended up with both a sore knee and a bruised ego.

As Yogi Berra said, "If you can't imitate him, don't copy him."

He also opined, "I really didn't say everything I said." So, take it for what it's worth.

Many gyms and yoga studios have free or discounted memberships for Medicare members or folks over 65, so check around for what's offered in your neighborhood. My local community center also has a nice gym that's free for residents plus a lot of different exercise classes from Tai Chi to Pickleball.

It can be frustrating when we come to realize that we can't do what was previously easy and fun for us. My brother-in-law used to run several miles every day until the daily pounding started tearing up his knees. So, he switched to biking. Now he's walking. He's covering the same ground– just a little slower.

George Burns knew all about this. He said, "You know you're getting old when you stoop to tie your shoes and wonder what else you can do while you're down there."

Many of us are concerned about the possibility of having Alzheimer's Disease - a condition that slowly robs us of our memory and other brain functions. The good news is that the Alzheimer's Research and Prevention Foundation found that regular physical exercise can even reduce your risk of developing the disease by up to 50%.

The key is consistency. Make exercise a non-negotiable part of your schedule, like brushing your teeth or calling your friends and family.

Posture Power

Good posture isn't just about looking poised, it's essential for overall health. Slouching puts undue stress on your spine, leading to aches, pains, and reduced lung capacity. Imagine your head as a helium balloon, gently pulling your spine upward. Sit up straight, roll your shoulders back, and engage your core. Your body will thank you.

I know all about this. My wife has great posture and I have lousy posture. She is constantly reminding me to sit up straight, tuck my chin in and suck in my gut. I know one day I will thank her. And every time I see an older person hunched over, I immediately straighten up because none of us want to end up looking straight at the ground instead of greeting the horizon.

Here are some simple exercises you can use to enhance your posture from the Aspire Senior Center in Cleveland:

Back to the Wall:

- Stand with your back against a wall.

- Ensure that the back of your head, shoulder

blades, hips, and the back of your legs all touch the wall.

- Use the wall as support to position your body flush against it. This exercise helps you become aware of your posture and encourages proper alignment.

Chin Tucks and Juts:

- Sit or stand comfortably.

- Gently tuck your chin toward your chest, lengthening the back of your neck.

- Then, gently jut your chin forward, maintaining a neutral spine.

- Repeat this movement to strengthen the neck muscles and improve neck alignment.

Wall Tilts:

- Stand with your back against a wall.

- Place your hands on the wall at shoulder height.

- Tilt your pelvis backward, engaging your gluteal muscles.

- Hold for a few seconds and release.

- This exercise strengthens the pelvis and gluteal muscles, promoting better posture.

Scapular Retractions:

- Sit or stand with your arms by your sides.

- Squeeze your shoulder blades together, pulling them toward your spine.

- Hold for a few seconds and release.

- Repeat to strengthen the upper back muscles and improve shoulder alignment.

Bird Dogs:

- Begin on your hands and knees (tabletop position).

- Extend your right arm forward and your left leg backward simultaneously.

- Keep your spine neutral and engage your core.

- Return to the starting position and switch sides.

- This exercise improves spinal stability and balance.

I also like using a foam roller. I lie on the floor with the roller directly under my spine and supporting my head. I can actually feel my neck and spine relaxing. I also use it to roll out my calves and IT band – the long muscle that stretches from the hip all the way down to the knees.

Remember to perform these exercises regularly and be mindful of your posture throughout the day. Consistency is key to maintaining good alignment and reducing aches and pains. And always check with your doctor or medical team before starting any new exercise routine.

Regular Check-Ups

Your medical team isn't just there for emergencies. Regular check-ups are like preventive maintenance for your body. Schedule annual visits with your primary care physician, dentist, and any specialists you need. Discuss your health goals, ask questions, and follow their advice.

Although they are the experts, you are the patient. You are in charge of your health. If you don't understand something, ask, ask, ask until you understand the issue and what solutions are being proposed.

Doctors need to treat patients with respect and listen to you, not treat you as just a Medicare number on a sheet. Your medical team must earn your trust before you can trust their guidance.

And if you really don't feel comfortable with your doctor or feel they are dismissing your symptoms, find a second opinion or another doctor! One who will actually listen to you.

Communication Is Key

Don't play hide-and-seek with your symptoms. If something feels off, speak up. Whether it's a persistent cough, joint pain, or unexplained fatigue, share it with your doctor. They can't help you if they don't know what's going on. Be honest about your lifestyle, stress levels, and any changes you've noticed. Together, you'll create a roadmap to better health.

I have several friends who were reluctant to ask their doctor about certain nagging health issues. They thought they weren't important or that the doctor was too busy to respond to such unimportant questions. One of them was fortunate to have a daughter who pressed her to speak up. And she discovered that her "little concern" was actually the symptom of arterial blockage. She ended up having a procedure that likely saved her life.

Aging brings challenges to our bodies and it's up to us to respond appropriately.

As I mentioned at the beginning of this chapter, your health is like a car and you are the driver. No one else is in charge but you. Keep it running like a champ.

By prioritizing movement, exercise, posture, sleep, and open communication with your medical team, you're investing in a future where you can savor life's moments — whether it's dancing at your grandchild's wedding or climbing a mountain at sunrise. So, lace up those sneakers, stand tall, sleep well, and let health be your lifelong companion.

Chapter 4
Seize The Day
Finish Any Unfinished Business

One of the great mysteries of life is that none of us know when our final day on the planet will come. Some want to avoid thinking about it while others become obsessed with it. The great Buddhist teacher Nichiren encouraged his followers to live each day as if it were their last.

Personally, my goal is to conclude my life with no regrets. So, let's explore how to seize the day, tie up loose ends, and make every moment count.

The Grudge-Free Zone

Remember that time Cousin Mildred borrowed your favorite teapot and returned it with a chip? Or when you loaned your nephew Jimmy $200 and he never paid you back? Or when your neighbor Harold borrowed your new lawn mower and it never worked right again? Well, it's time to release those grudges like helium balloons.

Forgiveness isn't just a gift to others – it's a liberating act for yourself.

Grudges are like negative energy that slowly eats away at you. They are a form of resentment that over time can turn into a fetid bloom of bitterness. Older people are often accused of being cranky curmudgeons, and grudges are one of the main causes.

Most of the time, grudges are based on miscommunication or misunderstandings between people. Someone didn't do what you thought they said they would do. Or they didn't respond to a call or email you sent. There might be a million reasons why they did what they did, but without good communication, we tend to assume the worst. This kind of thing can often be cleared up with a simple phone call, but instead it can fester for years growing from indignation to resentment.

Get rid of it. Let it go!

Sometimes you might have a legitimate reason for being frustrated. Maybe your bank imposed a bunch of fees without telling you, or a salesperson was rude to you, or you were taken advantage of by someone.

To my way of thinking, you have two simple choices:

1. Rectify the situation: ask for an explanation, request a review, file a complaint, or hire an attorney.

2. Let it go! Move on.

Most of us are carrying around resentments like a leaking bag of acid. The only person that bag is burning is us.

There's a story about two Buddhist monks who are traveling from one monastery to another under a vow of silence. They come to a wide river and need to cross. Sitting on the banks next to them is a woman. She, too, needs to cross, but she's anxious about crossing safely. Without saying a word, one of the monks picks up the woman and carries her across the river on his shoulders. The other monk is shocked, but they keep walking in silence. Finally, they arrive at their destination where they can break their vow of silence. The angry monk sputters, "Why did you pick up that woman?! You know it's against the rules of our order to touch women!"

The other monk replies, "I put her down hours ago. Why are you still carrying her around?"

I suggest you take a moment and think about anyone or anything you might be carrying around as resentment. You may not realize how much that resentment or disappointment has been weighing you down. Is it time to put down that heavy burden?

Here are a few suggestions:

Forgive But Don't Forget

Grab your pen or smartphone and compose a heartfelt letter. Tell Cousin Mildred that you have pardoned her from the teapot jail, Harold's lawn mower wreck is ancient history, and Jimmy's loan is forgiven.

Now, let me be clear: we are not absolving anyone of their responsibility. As all Buddhists know, the Law of Cause and Effect is strict. Anyone who makes a bad cause will get a negative effect...eventually. But like the monk in the story I shared, we don't want to be the one carrying around the heavy weight of resentment. So, by forgiving them we are clearing our plate of the negative emotions. We don't need to give Jimmy another loan or offer the lawn mower to any other neighbors, but we are making peace and letting them know.

Burn It

If you aren't ready to actually send a forgiveness letter to someone you believe may have wronged, disappointed, or taken advantage of you, that's ok. Write the letter anyway. Tell them exactly how their actions made you feel. And then, take the paper outside and light it on fire – safely! Watch it burn and imagine your resentment, hurt or disappointment going up in smoke.

If that doesn't work, you might take some small comfort in the wise words of one of my favorite philosophers, Groucho Marx, who said, "Time wounds all heels!"

There's another way of dealing with old hurts, disappointments and resentments and that is therapy. Just talking to someone who is on your side, but has no dog in this hunt can be very freeing. And there are so many excellent therapeutic methods these days including, Emotional Freedom Technique Tapping, Cognitive Behavioral Therapy, and even psychedelic assisted psychotherapy.

At one time there was a stigma attached to seeing a therapist. But no longer. People of all ages and backgrounds have found real help through therapy.

There is a therapist and a methodology that's right for you. And most Medicare options cover it! So please don't hesitate to find someone you can talk to.

Don't Wait for Them to Call — Call Anyway!

Forgiveness is one part of preparing your life for the inevitable. You can also start letting the people you love, who have been kind to you, or inspired you, know how you feel about them.

Life's too short for missed connections. If you're waiting for someone to call, stop tapping your foot and dial their number. Whether it's an old friend, estranged sibling, or the plumber who fixed your leaky faucet in '98, reach out:

- **The Reunion:** Call up an old friend or work colleague. Look up your high school sweetheart. Who knows? They might really get a kick out of your call.

- **The Thank You**: Call or write your first grade teacher. Thank them for teaching you to tie your shoelaces and dream big. Thank a coach, relative, or colleague who mentored you.

- **Tell Them You Love Them:** So many people never heard their parents tell them that they loved them. "It was understood, but not spoken," a friend told me. But in my book that's not good enough. Make the call. Tell your kids, grandkids, siblings, heck even the UPS man (maybe not the UPS man) that you love them. It can have a transformative effect on both you and them.

The Buddha always spoke first. Why? To break the ice. He knew most people are shy and don't know what to say. Be bold and make the first move – even if it's only after 47 years. Do it now!

The Procrastination Tango - Don't Put It Off

Procrastination is like a dance—two steps forward, three Netflix episodes back. So, let's tango with time:

1. **The Doctor's Visit**: That mole on your elbow? Get it checked. Maybe it's just a freckle, but better safe than sorry. This is so important that I will keep repeating it!

2. **The Bucket List**: Skydiving? Learning the ukulele? Don't wait for a cosmic sign—book

that tandem jump and strum those strings.

Get Your Affairs in Order

The time to write your will is while you are still in decent health. The time to determine who gets what when you're gone is now. Don't assume that your heirs will figure it out.

I've got news for you; if you don't draw up a will, the state will decide who gets your assets and possessions. And I don't know about you, but the last person I want divvying up my stuff is some bureaucrat in probate court.

I won't belabor this topic, because I know it's a sensitive one for many people. We all think we are going to live forever, but unfortunately, none of us will. The best time to buy insurance is when you don't need it. And the best time to plan for the unpleasant is while things are still OK.

Here's what you need - at a minimum:

1. **A Will** - Pick a trusted person to be your executor and then decide who gets what. Be generous and be fair. This is not the time to be punitive.

2. **A Medical Directive** - This tells your medical team and family what lengths you want them to go to in case you become incapacitated. This can include instructions for a DNR (Do Not Resuscitate) if your condition becomes irreversible.

3. **Medical Power of Attorney** - This is a document that appoints a trusted person to make medical decisions on your behalf if you become unable to make these decisions yourself. This is really important, because without it, most states will allow a doctor – who may be a complete stranger – to make life or death decisions for you.

4. **Family Trust** - If you have significant assets like property, stock, collections, patents or intellectual property, you should seriously consider putting them in a trust. Why? Because a will only prevents your estate from going into probate (state control) and expresses your wishes. But if you have significant assets, there can be real tax consequences for the transfer of your stuff to your heirs.

A good estate attorney can help you with all this. At the very least, please consider having a conversation about these topics with your kids, family members, or trusted friends. This is the best way to prepare for the unexpected.

Finish Unfinished Business

We all have unfinished business. If we want to live out our lives to the fullest with no regrets we have to own up to anything we know we need to take care of while we are still vertical.

There may be some things in our lives we need to set straight. If you need to correct the record on something, now is the time to write out your version of the story.

If you haven't told your kids, your grandkids, or your siblings that you love them, pick up the phone today.

If there's someone you want to reconnect with or express appreciation to, send them a note.

If you are carrying grudges or resentment towards people – living or deceased – seek ways to release it.

And if there's a secret that you need to reveal, a burden you don't want to take with you to the grave, decide who to tell it to and when. Deathbed confessions are something no one wants.

Wipe the slate clean. You'll feel a whole lot better when you do.

And do it now! Carpe diem!

Chapter 5
Spend Your Savings
It's Your Money

If you followed the advice most of us were given when we were younger, you have socked away some money for your retirement. But here's the thing, a lot of us won't really retire. More and more people over 65 continue to work – some of us because we have to, some because we don't want to sit on the porch all day.

Hey, there's nothing wrong with retirement, you earned it. But some people have squirreled away enough money to get to 120. At the same time, your expenses may have gone down; you aren't paying for 3 kid's college tuition and a mortgage and two car loans anymore. Between lower monthly expenses, savings, and a 401K or pension, many of us have more money than we will ever need.

"Wait a minute", you might be thinking. "My pension could evaporate. Social Security could go belly up. Banks could fail."

All true, but unlikely.

You might have had parents or grandparents who lived through the great depression. I did. They told stories about having to stretch canned food, sell newspapers for pennies, and go door to door looking for work. It was a terrible time for many.

A lot of them didn't have social security. We do.

Many didn't have pensions or 401K plans. We do.

No one wants to run out of money in their old age. But according to a Wharton-University of Pennsylvania study, the average person who passes away between the ages of 60-90 leaves behind an estate of around $300,000. That's $300K they didn't spend in their lifetime. And this doesn't take into account the 10% of US households who have a net worth over $1 million. They are likely to leave behind even more assets.

So, what should we do with this extra cash?

Professional retirement planners sometimes talk about the three stages of our senior years:

- The Go-Go years
- The Slow-Go years

- The No-Go years

What does this mean?

From ages 55-70 we may still have plenty of energy, interest, and gumption to travel, explore, bike, hike, ski, or kayak to our heart's content. We can trek across the great cities of Europe or endure a long flight to Asia and still be ready for more. These are our Go-Go years.

By the time we are in our 70s, many of us won't be as energetic or active as were just years before. We will get tired more easily, have more aches and pains, and medical conditions that may limit our mobility and stamina. We might not want to stay up all night on a flight to Europe or walk across the hard cobblestone streets of Paris, but instead book a shorter flight or choose a bus tour. We can still get out and enjoy the world, but this time in our lives is called the Slow-Go years because we need to take it easy.

If we are fortunate enough to reach 85, we might be entering our No-Go years.

This is the time when even if we wanted to trek across Europe, sail the high seas, or go back to Disney World, our bodies simply won't let us. Sure, there's the centenarian who runs marathons, but they are the exception that proves the rule.

So, here's the tricky part...

Why aren't we spending most of our retirement money while we can actually enjoy it? Why aren't we taking our family to our ancestral homeland or the Magic Kingdom and running around while we can still run around?

Frankly, it's because most of us are worried that we will run out of money and die broke.

It's a fact that most of us will spend more money on our healthcare in the last 12 months of our lives than the previous 10 years. That's because if we become hospitalized and require long-term care, the expenses can add up quickly.

Medicare, Medigap, or a combination of other insurance products can help cover these expenses. But even if you budget $100K for you and your spouse for your last year above and beyond Social Security, pensions, and Medicare, you may still reach the end of your life with money in the bank.

So why not enjoy it while you can?

In his book, Die With Zero, Bill Perkins provides an interesting take on this topic that I found really helpful. It's a thought-provoking framework for maximizing what he calls "net fulfillment" over net worth.

Perkins promotes the idea of both saving and spending. Rather than scrimping and saving every extra penny for our retirement, he recommends intentionally spending our hard-earned money on the things that bring us joy and fulfillment while we can still get the most out of them.

According to Perkins, traditional financial planning presses us to increase our net worth until we stop working, but by then many of us become afraid or unable to even enjoy it.

I agree with his basic premise that your life is the sum of your experiences. By investing in experiences, you unlock something he calls "memory dividends." Experiences yield dividends because we enjoy recounting our positive memories.

We've all heard about the changes in the way younger people feel about gifts. Instead of stuff, they want experiences. These experiences become part of the story of their lives.

By optimizing experiences, we can also get this memory dividend – that warm and fuzzy feeling we get recalling that trip to Mexico with our kids or the Airstream caravan to the Grand Canyon. Or even the subscription to the local theater.

I really like that Perkins teaches us how to trade money for something of greater value: moments of pure joy. These memories are our ultimate treasure.

This helped me understand that what I used to call a "splurge" is not really an extravagance. It's actually a way of enjoying my life today while creating memories I can dip into later in my life as well.

Old and Broke. Now What?

OK, great. But what if you don't have any savings, or you've been through a challenging health event that has drained your savings?

That's tough. And many of us will face unexpected challenges.

According to the US Census, there are 6 million people over 65 living below the poverty line in America today.

I'll be honest with you. My mom is one of them. She did not prepare well for her retirement and ran out of money in her 80s. But she is fortunate that my siblings and I have the means and the will to support her and provide for her now that she is in her 90s.

Social security alone is not enough for most of us to live on in retirement. That means if we haven't saved, we will be facing some difficult choices. We may have to sell our home or liquidate any assets or items of value we might still own.

These choices may be limited by our health as well.

Some of us will be working into our 80s to help make ends meet. Others will be reliant on generous relatives. And some of us will become wards of the state or private charities.

These are not happy options. If you are young(ish) and don't have much in savings, I hope that while you have the energy and mobility, you will think, plan, and act carefully to maximize your ability to support yourself in your Slow-Go and No-Go years.

AARP (the American Association of Retired People) has a bunch of resources to help you prepare for retirement. They also have a state-by-state directory of services that are available to you if you don't have the means to support yourself.

Spend? Save? Hoard cash? Splurge? There's no one solution for everyone. It all depends on your situation, your life expectancy, and your bank account.

Finding the balance between prudent planning and living life to the fullest is like a dance with steps that shift and tempos that change with the melody of your evolving circumstances. There's no right answer but having an open dialogue between your heart and your head can help you find the right path – the path to living a life of no regrets.

Chapter 6
Curious Minds Never Age

The Lifelong Learning Adventure

Many of us couldn't wait to get out of school and on with our lives. But as we now know, nothing is constant but change, especially in areas like health, science, and technology.

Researchers have discovered that learning isn't just for the young – it's the secret elixir for a vibrant life. It may not be the fountain of youth, but just as we can slow the impact of aging on our bodies, we now know we can do the same for our minds.

According to a recent AARP study on lifelong learning, 55% of Americans aged 45 and older are actively learning new things. Many are driven to seek personal growth and self-betterment as opposed to work and career advancement. The study found the most popular areas of interest were history, food and drink, mental health, technology, and nutrition.

So, let's embark on a lifelong learning adventure that will help keep our mind spry, our memory strong, and our brain active.

The Brain Gym

Picture this: You are sitting in a cozy armchair, sipping chamomile tea, and unraveling the mysteries of quantum physics. Okay, maybe not quantum physics, but you get the idea. So, what can we explore?

- **History**: Dive into the past like a time-traveling detective. Unravel ancient civilizations, decipher hieroglyphics, and impress your grandkids with tales of Cleopatra's cat collection.

- **Music**: Dust off that old guitar or pick up a ukulele. Learning an instrument keeps your brain humming and your soul singing. Join a choir or vocal group and harmonize.

- **Cooking**: Knead dough, whip up soufflés, and become a culinary maestro. Bonus points if you can explain the science behind a perfectly risen soufflé.

Lifelong Learning in the Digital Age

- YouTube **University:** Remember when VHS tapes ruled the world? Well, now it's YouTube's turn. Want to learn watercolor painting? All of Bob Ross' old TV shows are on Youtube. Building a greenhouse? There's a tutorial for that. Curious about astrophysics? Neil deGrasse Tyson awaits. YouTube is one of our primary digital classrooms. It's free, accessible, and entertaining–just don't get distracted by all the cat videos.

- Khan Academy**:** Created in 2006 by Sal Khan as a way to help his young cousin learn math, Khan Academy is an education non-profit that has produced over 10,000 instructional video lessons covering a dizzying array of academic subjects, including mathematics, biology, literature, history, and computer science. Their videos are used by students all around the world, including lifelong learners. After being in the dark for years, I finally learned how to solve an equation for X–at the same time an 8 year old in India was learning it! I love Khan Academy.

The Social Symphony

Learning doesn't have to be a solo act. There are so many opportunities to learn and share with others.

The Book Club Bonanza: During the pandemic, membership in book clubs skyrocketed as a way of creating connection while we were all stuck at home. Now that the dreaded virus is on its hind leg, book clubs are meeting in person again as well as online. Both good places to start. Some local libraries also sponsor book clubs as do many senior and community centers. Whether you love mysteries, fantasy, or medieval history, there's a club for you. Discuss great literature, sip herbal tea (or something stronger), and forge friendships that rival the best novel endings.

Finish College in Outer Space: OK, not quite yet, but many universities offer continuing or community education courses in person and online. You can even get credit to help complete that degree in underwater basket weaving – or maybe not. Coursera.com and AARP.org are good places to start.

Tech Tango: No matter how you feel about smartphones, tablets, and other digital devices, they are here to stay. And every year the designers and programmers load on more features, functions, and doo-hickeys that drive many of us crazy. Not to mention the unwanted automatic upgrades, paywalls, and occasional hacks. It's enough to make you want to throw your phone in the toilet. Don't do it though, it's both expensive and embarrassing...take it from me.

We all need to have at least a minimal familiarity with current technology. It's hard to stay in contact with our friends and family if we don't understand video calling, Facetime, or texting.

And yes, it's probably true that just when you start to get the hang of these things they will get changed, upgraded, or even terminated. That's just the way of technology nowadays.

Don't Be A Tech Victim

We also need to be savvy enough to avoid being hacked, exploited, or having our data stolen. Having a computer, email program or online bank account that doesn't at least have two-factor authentication – one step more than just a password – is just as bad as leaving your wallet or purse on the dashboard of your unlocked car. It's an invitation for bad people to make you miserable.

Online, digital, and cyber protection is beyond the scope of this book, so I urge you to find a trusted 16-year-old who can help you understand how to secure your devices, back up your data, and identify bad actors.

Here's my absolute minimum set of tech "nevers:"

- Never give your passwords to a stranger for any reason

- Never allow a stranger to use your phone or computer

- Never click on links that come in emails - unless you're sure it's from a legit source

- Never, ever, send or wire money to anyone for any reason if solicited via email. Even if they are claiming to be a friend or family member in trouble

- And remember, no Nigerian prince is holding a fortune for you!

Let's be lifelong learners – curious, open-minded, and forever young at heart.

Whether you're deciphering hieroglyphics, strumming a ukulele, or baking soufflés, remember: growing old may stink sometimes, but learning? That's our golden ticket to a life well-lived. After all, curiosity doesn't age – it just gets wiser.

Chapter 7
Snooze or Lose
Sleep Like a Pro

As seasoned snoozers, we've earned the right to slumber like royalty. So, fluff those pillows, dim the lights, and let's explore how to catch those elusive Zs with style and grace.

As we age, we need more sleep. But it can also be harder to fall asleep and stay asleep. Personally, I consider it a good night if I only get up to go to the bathroom once.

Tests show that many of us just aren't producing the same amount of melatonin and serotonin as we did when we were younger. These are the hormones that tell our body it's time to shut down for some shut eye.

Studies have linked bad sleep to all kinds of health problems including higher levels of beta-amyloid in the brain, a metabolic waste product found in the fluid between neurons. When it clumps together, the clusters form amyloid plaques which halt communication between brain cells. In other words, poor sleep causes a protein buildup in your brain that, over time, increases memory loss and cognitive impairment and is directly linked to higher likelihood of developing Alzheimer's Disease.

Yikes! If that's not a good enough reason to prioritize sleep, you might also want to know that poor sleep impacts our decision-making ability, driver safety, and sexual functions.

If you are experiencing any of the symptoms of sleep deprivation or just want to have a more restful night's sleep, here are several things for you to consider.

Reduce Caffeine intake

This one might seem obvious to you, but many of us are so hooked on our morning coffee we forget that as we age, it takes longer for your body to work off the effects of this stimulant. Black tea has less caffeine, but still enough to have an impact. It can take up to 12 hours before the effects of coffee or black tea wear off. That means if you have a cup of joe at lunch you could be setting yourself up for some unwanted night owl time.

I am extra sensitive to caffeine so I stick to decaf coffee, even in the mornings. But I'm also a chocoholic and there's plenty of hidden caffeine in my favorite sweet treat – especially dark chocolate, which can have as much caffeine in it as black tea. After learning this, I switched to eating my chocolate in the morning.

Hey mom, I'm a grown up! I can eat dessert whenever I want!

Stick to the Sleep Schedule

Remember when time was a loose concept, and bedtime was negotiable? Well, those days are over. You have to stick to a regular sleep schedule. Go to bed and rise at the same time every day – even on weekends. Consistency helps regulate your internal clock and ensures smoother transitions between dreamland and reality.

Create a Bedtime Ritual

Develop a soothing bedtime routine. Think of it as your personal lullaby. Here's an example:

- **Dim the Lights**: Like a theater before the show, lower the lights at least 30 minutes before bedtime. Your brain will get the memo, "Curtains closing soon."

- **Screen Detox**: Bid adieu to screens (yes, even YouTube and TikTok) at least an hour before bed. Blue light messes with your melatonin production – the hormone responsible for sleepiness. You might even consider moving your TV out of your bedroom. It can help with screen detox, and might even improve your love life!

- **Have a Cup of Calming Tea**: Sip on chamomile, lavender or valerian tea—it's like a warm hug for your insides. Each of these varieties are known to help relax the body and mind.

- **Consider Sleep Aids**: If calming teas don't do the trick, talk with your doctor or medical team about over the counter and prescription sleep aids. My body does well with a small amount of melatonin, but my wife needs something stronger. Or you could do what our Irish friend does and have a wee dram of whiskey right before bed. He says it helps him sleep like a baby.

The Bedroom Oasis

Your bedroom should be a sanctuary—a cocoon of tranquility. Here's how to create the ultimate sleep haven:

- **Cool and Dark**: As we age, we become more sensitive to light, so channel your inner bat. Keep the room cool (around 65°F) and pitch-dark. You might invest in some blackout curtains – they're like superhero capes for shut-eye.

- **Comfy Mattress**: Your mattress should be as supportive as a loyal friend. If it's sagging like a deflated balloon, consider an upgrade.

- **Consider a Mattress Warmer**: There's nothing worse than climbing into an ice cold bed in winter. We love our mattress warmer. It not only keeps us cozy and warm on chilly nights, it also helps with circulation.

- **White Noise**: If the neighbor's dog moonlights as a midnight opera singer, drown out the noise with a white noise machine. Ah, blissful silence.

Meditate Your Way to Dreamland

Far and away the simplest and least expensive method to fall asleep is meditation. Meditation in this case is just the simple repetition of certain phrases that stop the incessant yammering of your mind and tell your body that it's time to sleep. There are many examples available on YouTube or sites like Headspace.com and Reveri.com.

Here are a few that I really like:

- **Three Deep Breaths**: My friend En-May Mangels, a world-renowned intuitive, teaches this to her clients. It calms the mind and puts you in a state of gratitude and appreciation. Start by getting into bed and lying on your back. Take three slow, deep breaths. The first deep breath is for all the gifts of the past. We have all received so many gifts in our lives. The second deep breath is for all the gifts of the present. What is alive with gratitude for you in this moment. And the third deep breath is for all the gifts that have yet to come. Now return to breathing normally.

- **Repeat a simple mantra**: A mantra is a phrase you say over and over in your mind that can help you enter a relaxed state. I like "deep relaxation." As I breathe in, I say to myself the word "deep," and as I breathe out, I say "relaxation." By the time I've done this four or five times I'm usually drifting off to sleep.

- **Hip Yourself to Self-Hypnosis**: This one really helped me when I was waking up in the middle of the night and having trouble getting back to the business of bagging more Zs. I repeat the following to myself: "I am getting sleepy, drowsy, my eyelids are becoming heavy. I'm falling into a deep, relaxing sleep from which I will wake up at 7 am in the morning, alert and awake having had a healing, rejuvenating night's sleep." Just writing this makes me drowsy!

Avoid the Nap Trap

Napping is like a tempting siren, luring you into its cozy embrace. But beware! Afternoon naps can sabotage your nighttime slumber. I love a good nap myself, but I've learned if you gotta nap, keep it short (20–30 minutes) and preferably before 3pm. Otherwise, you might find yourself wide-eyed at 2 am, pondering the mysteries of the universe or cursing the darkness.

Let's embrace our sleep like a cherished heirloom. Remember, you're not a nocturnal owl – just a wise, old owl. So, tuck in, count imaginary sheep, and drift into dreamland. Sweet dreams, my fellow starlit travelers!

Chapter 8

Write Your Memoirs - Throw A Pre-Memorial Party

Ah, the golden years – the time when life's wrinkles become laugh lines, and our memories are like a well-worn book with dog-eared pages. Through the years, we've accumulated tales that deserve to be shared, celebrated, and immortalized. So, grab your favorite pen (or tablet) and let's dive into the world of memoirs, stories, and pre-memorial parties!

Write Your Memoirs

Remember the days when typewriters clacked and inkwells were standard classroom equipment? (OK, maybe not the inkwells part, but I did love my old IBM Selectric.) Well, dust off your quill (or open your laptop) because it's time to write your memoirs. Here's how:

- **Choose Your Angle**: Are you the adventurous globetrotter, the culinary connoisseur, or the neighborhood gossip? Pick an angle that resonates with you.

- **Start with Snippets**: Don't stress about writing chronologically. Begin with snippets—a childhood memory, a quirky neighbor, or that time you accidentally dyed your hair neon green.

- **Be Honest**: Memoirs thrive on authenticity. Share your triumphs, mistakes, your brushes with greatness and loss.

- **Edit with Love**: Write, write, and then write some more. Then like pruning a rosebush, trim unnecessary details. Your memoirs should sparkle, not overwhelm.

The Joy of Reminiscing

As you write, let nostalgia sweep you away. This is the one time you can really live in the past. Recall the smell of grandma's freshly baked oatmeal raisin cookies, the thrill of your first bicycle ride, and the taste of victory when you finally beat your middle school nemesis at Pac-Man. Your memoirs are a gift to future generations—a time capsule of wisdom, wit, and whimsy.

Ok, let's say you're not so good at writing or typing. No problem. Try idea #2...

The Art of Oral Tradition

Gather your family and friends (or anyone who will listen!) around the proverbial fireside (or actual fireplace if you're feeling cozy). It's storytime! Share your tales of resilience, love, and the Great Sock Puppet Incident of '72. Remember:

- **Characters Matter**: Introduce Aunt Mildred, the knitting champion who once unraveled a mystery using yarn. Spill the beans about your first high school girlfriend who later came out as gay. Just keep it G rated - kids may be listening.

- **Add Drama**: Embellish a tad. Turn a minor mishap into an epic adventure involving lost treasure and a mischievous squirrel. As one great writer shared, never let the facts get in the way of a good story.

- **Laughter Is the Best Glue**: Stories bind us.

Chuckles and guffaws create lasting bonds. Share your favorite practical jokes, riddles, and limericks.

- **Record everything on your phone or voice recorder.** Today there are so many inexpensive transcription services, there's no need to write it all out. Don't worry, they can edit out all the "ums" and "uhs."

The Wisdom Circle

Invite a few fellow gray beards for a storytelling soirée. Gather in a sunlit room, sip chamomile tea or an adult beverage, and take turns sharing snippets from your lives. The best part? No judgment—only snaps, applause, and knowing nods.

Here are some prompts to help you get the ball rolling:

- What was your greatest moment in high school or college?
- What was the biggest mistake you ever made on a job?
- Who had the greatest impact on you as a

child?

- What was your best and worst family vacation?

- Which teacher or coach helped you the most?

- What was your worst date?

- How did you meet your spouse?

Hint: have someone record this session with their phone or video camera.

Throw a Pre-Memorial Party

Don't be like Garrison Keillor who said, "They say such nice things about people at their funerals that it makes me sad to realize that I'm going to miss mine by just a few days."

Instead, bask in the warmth, the love, the joy of seeing and being with loved ones. Send out whimsical invites: "Join Us for a Pre-Memorial Shindig!" Include a disclaimer: "No Eulogies Allowed." Encourage guests to wear period costumes or their quirkiest hats or colorful socks. No black suits or dresses! Provide snacks and refreshments suitable for adults and kids, if invited.

The Activities

- **Life Timeline**: String up a clothesline and hang photos representing different life stages. Let guests reminisce and guess which decade each snapshot belongs to.

- **Speech:** Welcome and thank everyone for coming. Then invite others to come up and share stories about your lives together. Be prepared though, these events sometimes turn into hilarious roasts of the guest of honor, so take it all in with grace and aplomb. Invite those who can't attend in person to record a short message.

- **Legacy Wall**: Set up a wall where guests can write heartfelt messages or share their favorite memories of you.

- **Record Everything**: Have someone record the event. If there's time, ask each attendee to record a memory or sentiment. Take my word for it, you will cherish these recordings later.

The Last Toast

As the host, raise your glass and propose a toast. You can write your own or use George Burns': "To all my old friends, and nobody has friends older than I do."

Or you can say something like, "To life, laughter, and the joy of being gloriously alive!"

Let's weave our stories, ink our memoirs, record our victories and challenges, and most of all, let's dance at our pre-memorial parties. Life is a grand adventure, and we are the seasoned explorers. So, my dear friend, gather your loved ones, tell your tales, and celebrate—you've earned it!

Chapter 9

Simplify, Clear Out, And Release

Let Go of Unnecessary Stuff

As we journey through the various stages of life, we can accumulate a staggering amount of stuff. Everything from souvenirs collected during travels, to unwanted gifts like the singing Big Mouth Billy Bass–not to mention those impulse buys we thought would bring us joy but now sit gathering dust.

This accumulation can easily start to feel overwhelming, even suffocating. But fear not! Simplifying and clearing out our physical space can bring a sense of liberation and joy. The Buddha loved simplicity so let's declutter not just our homes, but our minds as well.

Simplicity Can Be Hard

The Buddha taught that attachment is one of the roots of human suffering. Our possessions, while sometimes useful and meaningful, can become burdens when we develop unhealthy attachments to them. I mean, how many salt shakers, golf clubs, or beanie babies does a person need?

Apparently, a lot.

I don't believe this concept of practicing non-attachment means we should renounce all worldly possessions and live like half-naked ascetics in a windowless cabin in the mountains, but rather, we should strive to find balance.

By simplifying our lives and reducing our physical clutter, we can cultivate a sense of peace and clarity.

Full disclosure: I am a collector. I collect all kinds of things, big and small. I love old fountain pens and pocket watches and pianos. Yep, the big wood ones with 88 keys. I own seven of them! Why? Because I like them!

But what's the difference between being a collector and a hoarder? Hoarding is a condition of compulsively accumulating things – oftentimes things that other people might consider worthless – and then being unable to discard anything without experiencing major distress.

Hoarding is a serious psychological condition. If you or someone you love has stuffed their home so full of stuff that you can't conduct daily life activities like cooking, entertaining, or just moving easily from room to room, then please seek professional help.

Collecting, on the other hand, is about the joy of finding, studying, sharing, and surrounding yourself with things that you love. At least a third of us collect something – snow globes, teddy bears, fossils, rare books, movie posters, model trains – the list is practically endless.

Another way to put it is that collecting things brings us joy, whereas hoarding is about the fear of letting go.

That said, most of us could use some pruning of our stuff. So, let's dive in…

The Real Benefits of Simplifying and Decluttering

- **Mental Clarity**: A cluttered space often leads to a cluttered mind. When you clear out unnecessary items, you create a calmer, more focused environment. This can lead to improved mental clarity and reduced stress.

It's like mental floss for your mind.

- **Increased Energy**: Physical clutter can drain your energy. By removing excess stuff, you create a more invigorating space, allowing you to feel more energized and motivated. Plus think of all the calories you'll burn humping all your junk to Goodwill or the Salvation Army.

- **Greater Freedom:** The fewer possessions you have, the less tied down you feel. This sense of freedom can be incredibly liberating, like a huge weight off your shoulders, allowing you to focus on experiences and relationships rather than material goods.

- **Enhanced Creativity**: A clean, organized space can foster creativity. Without the distraction of clutter and the guilty feelings that sometimes come with it, your mind is free to wander and explore new ideas.

- **Improved Well-being**: A tidy, organized home can lead to a greater sense of well-being. It can reduce anxiety and promote a sense of control over your environment.

Saying goodbye to stuff you don't need can be liberating. It can change the look, feel, and even the safety of your home. Getting rid of excess possessions is also a way of contributing to the welfare of others. Whether you donate to a charity, a family in need, or offer your stuff on one of the many local giveaway websites, you will be making a good cause. And who doesn't want to collect more karmic brownie points?

Steps to Simplify, Clear Out, and Release

Start Small: Tackling your entire home at once can be overwhelming. Begin with one small area, such as a single drawer or a corner of a room. If you are adventurous, you can pick a closet to start with, but don't start with something too overwhelming like your attic, basement, or a garage. This makes the process more manageable and less intimidating.

Set Clear Goals: Define what you want to achieve with your decluttering efforts. Are you looking to create more space, reduce stress, or simply live more minimally? Having clear goals will guide your actions and keep you motivated.

Create Categories: For your first pass, I recommend you sort your belongings into only two categories: "keep" or "goodbye." Once you've gone through your closet or dresser, put everything back that you plan to keep. Be honest with yourself about what you truly need and what you can let go of.

Now look at the outbound pile. Decide whether you want to donate, sell, or discard each item. Good clothing or home goods can be sold on Craigslist, eBay or to stores like CrossRoadsTrading.co. If you don't want the hassle of selling your items, you can donate them to charity or even just put them out on the curb with a sign that reads "FREE STUFF."

Ask the Right Questions: When deciding whether to keep an item, ask yourself:

- Does this bring me joy?

- Have I used this in the past year?

- Is this something I truly need?

- Could someone else benefit from this more?

Letting Go of Sentimental Items: Sentimental items can be the hardest to part with. Ask yourself which are the most meaningful pieces. Do I need five drawings from my kid's 3rd grade art class or an entire book of grandma's old wedding photos? Decide which tug most at your heartstrings and let go of the rest. I also suggest that you take photos of items to preserve the memories. That frees you up to release the physical object and hold onto only the most meaningful ones.

Adopt a One-In, One-Out Rule: To prevent future clutter, adopt the one-in, one-out rule. For every new item you bring into your home, let go of an existing one. Honestly, as a collector, I hate this one. But I have to admit it's generally good advice. Just don't tell my wife I said so.

Mindful Consumption: Moving forward, practice mindful consumption. Before making a purchase, consider if the item is truly necessary and if it aligns with your values and goals.

This is really the forward-looking component of everything we've just discussed. There will always be shiny new gadgets, doohickeys, and other products clamoring for our attention. Some of them will actually improve our lives and we shouldn't hesitate to add them to our inventory. But a lot of them won't really provide much joy or utility over time, so ask yourself twice: a year from now, will I be glad that I bought this? If not, leave it on the shelf.

Goodbye and Good luck

Releasing possessions can be incredibly freeing. It's a practice of non-attachment and letting go of the past. It can also be a way to give back. Donating items to those in need can bring joy to others and a sense of fulfillment to yourself.

But If decluttering feels overwhelming, seek support from friends, family, or even professional organizers. Sometimes an outside perspective can be incredibly helpful.

For a good place to start, I recommend Marie Kondo's book, The Life Changing Magic of Tidying Up. During the pandemic, a lot of us felt cooped up in our homes and Kondo's bestseller helped us use the time proactively to sort through all our stuff.

She asked us to pose a simple question when deciding whether or not to keep something: "Does this spark joy?" If it doesn't, then goodbye! So simple, yet it cuts to the heart of our attachments with things.

I have a friend who realized all her stuff was starting to make her feel heavy. She needed to change something, but where to start? She realized that if she kept her desk free of stacked papers, bills and magazines and her kitchen sink free of dirty dishes, that she could start to breathe easier. And it wasn't too hard to make steps from there to her bedroom and other areas.

Shred Your Schedule

Decluttering isn't just about physical items; it's also about simplifying your schedule. As we age, it's essential to prioritize activities that bring us joy and fulfillment.

Evaluate Commitments: Assess your current commitments and identify which ones truly add value to your life. Let go of those that don't. Don't let someone guilt you into committing to something you really don't want to do. Learn to say "no thanks," politely but firmly. It's okay to protect your time and energy.

Prioritize Self-Care: Make self-care a priority. This includes physical, mental, and emotional health. Schedule regular activities that nurture your well-being like gathering with friends, going out in nature, or getting massages.

Create Routines: Establishing daily and weekly routines can help simplify your life and reduce decision fatigue. Routines provide structure and predictability, which can be comforting and stabilizing. It also helps to remember that Monday is meatloaf, Tuesday is bowling, Wednesday is full of woe – just kidding! Just seeing if you were still paying attention!

The Spiritual Side of Simplifying Your Life

In Buddhism, the practice of simplification is closely tied to mindfulness. When we simplify our lives, we create more space to be present. We can appreciate the beauty in the ordinary moments and find joy in simplicity.

Declutter Your Mind: Approach decluttering as a mindfulness practice. Be fully present as you sort through your belongings, paying attention to the feelings and memories they evoke.

Have a Gratitude Practice: As you let go of items, practice gratitude for the role they played in your life. This can make the process more positive and less about loss. I have learned that I don't always need to keep pictures or mementos of people who have passed because I can keep them in my heart.

Breath and Look Within: I'm a big believer in meditation. It doesn't take much to get you out of all the mind chatter that goes on in our heads all the time. Just a few minutes of focusing on your breathing can be enough. There are many videos and apps that feature scores of meditations. I like Reveri.com but others like Headspace.com and Calm.com are also good. Meditation has been proven to help clear mental clutter and provide a sense of calm and clarity.

Connect with Nature: Go outside, every day if possible. Regardless of the weather, I get out every day and walk, hike, or bike. It helps that we have a dog who seems to have a 90 minute bladder limit. But even if you don't have a pet pulling at you for a walk, you can spend time in nature. You can reconnect with the simplicity of the natural world. Nature has a way of reminding us of what's truly important.

Embracing the Joy of Less

The process of simplifying and decluttering can lead to a profound sense of joy and contentment. By letting go of excess, we make room for what truly matters: meaningful relationships, personal growth, and inner peace.

Here are a couple of more thoughts to consider in order to maximize joy, fulfillment and satisfaction in your life:

Focus on Experiences: Prioritize experiences over possessions. Even inveterate collectors like me know this is true. Stuff comes and goes, but we've learned that experiences pay a memory dividend that can't be erased. A great meal with friends, a game of checkers with our grandkids, or a walk in the park are often more fulfilling than any material goods.

Cultivate Contentment: Learn to be content with what you have. This doesn't mean you shouldn't strive for better, but rather appreciate the present moment and your current blessings. I often reflect on how fortunate I am to have so much cool stuff. These things don't make me happy. Stuff can't make you happy. But art, antiques, books, snow globes, model trains, whatever it is – can bring you joy. And we can all use more joy in our lives.

I had a friend who collected antique and classic cars. At one point he owned 33 of them! The cost and hassle of garaging, maintaining, and just keeping track of all of them started to weigh him down. Then one day he told me he was going to sell them all (except for two he really loved). When I asked him why he replied, "Because I realized that with all those cars, I didn't really own them, they were starting to own me. And that wasn't working for me."

Simplifying, clearing out, and releasing excess stuff is more than just a practical task; it's a pathway to greater joy and freedom. By embracing the Buddhist principles of non-attachment and mindfulness, we can create a life that is rich in meaning and contentment. So, take a deep breath, roll up your sleeves, and begin the journey of simplifying your life. Remember, it's not just about getting rid of stuff; it's about making space for what truly matters.

Chapter 10

One is the Loneliest Number

Don't Go Solo

We've all heard about the epidemic of loneliness. So, if you are feeling alone, well, you're not alone.

We all need to have frequent and consistent interaction with others.

The U.S. Surgeon General, Dr. Vivek Murthy, has reported that lacking connection can increase the risk for premature death to levels comparable to smoking 15 cigarettes a day! His study found that even before the COVID-19 pandemic, about half of U.S. adults reported experiencing measurable levels of loneliness.

The Surgeon General warned that the physical consequences of poor connection can be devastating: 29% increased risk of heart disease, 32% increased risk of stroke, and a 50% increased risk of developing dementia for older adults.

Yikes! Growing old is hard enough, being alone while you're doing it is no fun.

There are many reasons we might find ourselves feeling lonely at this point in our lives. Kids get married, have families, and move away. Friends and spouses pass away or lose mobility. And frankly, many of us had social lives that revolved around our work. So, once we retired, we suddenly found ourselves with a lot of time on our hands and not many people to spend it with.

Dr. Murthy said loneliness isn't a uniquely American problem, rather it's a feature of modern life all around the globe. But, he noted that in the U.S. participation in community organizations - from faith groups to recreational leagues - has declined in recent decades.

If you are feeling lonely, the first thing to do is admit that you're feeling lonely!

That can be hard for some people. But there are ways to increase our connections to others and cure the aching heart of loneliness.

So, let's explore some potential solutions…

Community Gathering Programs

Senior center programming: These centers offer a variety of activities, classes, and social events for older adults. It's a great way to connect with peers and engage in hobbies.

"But I don't want to hang out with a bunch of old people," I was telling myself when this was suggested to me. "Dad, Get Over it!" my daughter insisted. And she was right, there are some wonderful people to meet right in your local community. Check it out.

Social adult day care: If you need assistance, these programs can provide supervised activities, meals, and social interaction for older adults during the day. Many of them also arrange or provide transportation so you don't have to worry about driving or taking public transportation

Congregate meals: Joining group meals at churches, community centers or senior centers can foster social connections. There are also group cooking programs that meet at community centers and even private homes. And believe it or not, sometimes the food is great - because it's cooked with love.

Volunteer opportunities: Volunteering provides you with an opportunity to contribute to your community while building relationships. It's a way to give back and connect at the same time. Many organizations are hungry for helpful people just like you to volunteer.

I volunteer at the Ballard Food Bank in Seattle. I bag groceries for our neighbors in need, but I also spend a lot of time kibitzing (chatting) with my fellow volunteers and staff. It feels like a second home for me and many of our clients have become regulars. I'm not the world's greatest bagger, but I know I'm doing something that really has meaning for me, our organization and our community. So be a hero in your community and try volunteering.

Who's Calling?

Friendly visiting programs: Many social service organizations provide volunteers to visit you at home, providing companionship and conversation. This may sound odd or even uncomfortable, to have a stranger come to your home. But legitimate organizations who provide home visits qualify their volunteers. Many churches, synagogues and other faith groups also provide home visits from clergy members or volunteers from their congregations.

Friendly calls programs: If you aren't comfortable welcoming someone new into your home you can try this program which provides regular phone calls from volunteers. Even a phone call with a stranger can combat loneliness. I had an uncle who used to call 411 - remember when telephones companies had live operators? Just to chat with someone.

Meals on Wheels: We've all heard about Meals On Wheels. This wonderful program serves over 2 million seniors every year and is hosted by over 5000 community organizations that deliver nutritious food to people who have food insecurity in all 50 states. Many of the volunteers provide regular conversation, friendship, and engagement with the people they deliver to. And it's free. If you have a car and a willingness to serve, you can be a volunteer too.

Technology and Digital Solutions

Online communities: OK, full disclosure, I really dislike Facebook. But it has become the #1 online meeting platform for people to find others who share their interests. It's my first stop when I want to learn more about a new hobby travel destination. Of course there are other virtual communities, forums, and social media platforms you can participate in as well.

Video calls: My dad learned how to use Zoom during the pandemic when he turned 90 so you can too. Regular video chats with family and friends can bridge physical distances. I really prefer seeing friends and family members' faces than just hearing their voices. Plus I can see if they are keeping their house clean – just kidding, but I am paying attention…

Digital classes and workshops: Learning new skills online can be both educational and socially engaging. There are lots of online classes that are pre-recorded and those can be educational, but if you want interaction I suggest you look up your local community college and see if their online courses offer something you'd find interesting or stimulating.

Pets to the Rescue

Research has shown us that possessing a companion animal can lead to a number of positive health outcomes – a phenomenon that has been called the "pet effect" previously. Pet owners had lower levels of frailty and higher levels of physical activity. In addition, pet ownership was shown to be related to lower levels of depressive symptoms and anxiety.

Pets can help connect us with our neighbors. A study in Australia found that pet owners are more likely to talk with people living in their neighborhood than non-pet owners. That makes sense as pet owners are always asking each other about their animals, food choices, vets, and so on.

Surprisingly, pets can not only help lower your stress level, another study even revealed that pet ownership was associated with higher likelihoods of survival after cardiovascular events – like strokes and heart attacks!

Adopt A Grand Dog

For some people owning a pet is not a problem. The tasks associated with feeding, walking and caring for a pet are well within their abilities. But what if you just aren't up to all that? Consider adopting a "Grand Dog." Find a local family with a loving pet they are willing to share with you. You can play with the dog, walk the dog, sit with it, and then just like actual grandparents, leave the messy part to the parents! This is a new concept so it might sound strange to some. But many pet owners could use a little help with walking, dog sitting or even contributing towards food and vet costs and might welcome your involvement. Just don't dress your grand dog in any weird outfits!

Loneliness is all around us. In a National Public Radio interview, the Surgeon General went on to talk about how insidious loneliness can be. "And you can feel lonely even if you have a lot of people around you, because loneliness is about the quality of your connections."

In my experience loneliness and depression are two sad bedfellows. Once you start feeling alone it's easy to get discouraged and start losing hope. If you are feeling lonely, please don't hesitate to reach out to someone. There are many free mental health programs for seniors on the local, county and state level. You can find someone in your neck of the woods at SAMSA.orgwhich provides a national directory of service providers.

Now, I want to tell you one of my favorite stories about connection. It was told to me by Dr. Bernie Siegal whose book helped jump start the self-healing and patient rights movements. Anyway, Bernie was telling me of a time he was asked to give a speech to some very uninterested high school kids at an inner-city school.

Standing on stage, he surveyed his audience and realized his prepared words were likely irrelevant to his audience. So he scrapped his speech and started with a surprising request. He asked the kids, "How many of you don't have a father at home?" Reluctantly many of the kids raised their hands.

"Take down this number," he instructed, and then read off seven digits.

"Everyone needs a father, so if you don't have one, now I'm your Dad." He continued, "You got a problem, you get in a jam, you need someone to talk to, call me. Call Dad."

The kids were stunned. So was I when I heard the story. Bernie told me he got a few calls like, "Hey Dad it's my birthday, where's my present?" But mostly it was just kids who needed someone to talk to. Someone with a compassionate and unbiased set of ears who could give them some good advice on challenges they were facing.

So, I'll make you the same deal. The truth is that it takes time to get connected to people in your local community or even online. So if you start feeling a bit down or lonely and need a friendly person to talk to then here's my number - 858 480 7703.

Yep, that is a real number of mine so don't call me at 4 am pacific if you can avoid it. Just introduce yourself and say you read my book and want to chat. And we will.

Remember, fostering social connections is essential for overall well-being. Whether through face-to-face interactions or online or Zoom, you can take proactive steps to combat social isolation and loneliness.

Chapter 11
Seek Beauty, Model Kindness, Accept Grace
Live Vibrantly Now

By now I think we can agree that growing old ain't easy. Or as my pessimistic friend used to say, "Life's a bitch and then you die." No wonder he had trouble keeping any friends.

Regardless of life's twists and turns, growing older doesn't have to be an endless burden. So much depends on our attitude.

Buddhist philosopher Daisaku Ikeda wrote, "It is important to maintain a vibrant, progressive spirit... All too often people lose the drive to move ahead as they grow older. But the decision to draw back or to take a step forward hinges on only a slight difference in one's attitude or resolve. In the final chapter of our life, however, that slight difference can have momentous consequences."

So how can we keep moving forward with such a vibrant, progressive spirit? I suggest that you integrate three core values into your daily life:

- Seek Beauty

- Model Kindness

- Accept Grace

Seek Beauty

In the hustle and bustle of everyday life, it's easy to overlook the beauty that surrounds us. But seeking beauty isn't just about appreciating the aesthetic; it's about finding joy in the ordinary and the extraordinary. As we age, our senses and perceptions might change, but our ability to appreciate beauty can grow even deeper.

Start by taking a moment each day to notice something beautiful. It could be a sunrise, the laughter of a grandchild, the taste of your favorite tea, or the rustle of leaves in the wind. Beauty is everywhere if we take the time to look for it. By actively seeking out these moments, we remind ourselves that life, despite its challenges, is filled with wonder.

In Buddhism, this practice of intentional observation is akin to the concept of mindfulness. It's about being present and fully engaging in the world around us with our eyes wide open. When we seek beauty, we are practicing mindfulness, grounding ourselves in the present moment, and finding joy in the here and now.

Moreover, seeking beauty can be a creative endeavor. Engaging in activities such as painting, gardening, arranging flowers, or even setting a table can be incredibly fulfilling. These activities not only allow us to create beauty but also to connect with our inner selves and express our emotions in a positive and constructive way.

Consider keeping a journal where you note down moments of beauty you encounter each day. This practice can serve as a reminder of the positivity and goodness in the world, even on days when it feels hard to find. Over time, this habit can cultivate a more optimistic and appreciative outlook on life.

Model Kindness

Kindness is a universal virtue that transcends age, culture, and time. As we grow older, we can become cranky— sometimes without realizing it. Cast off the curmudgeon and choose kindness instead.

Modeling kindness can become a profound way to influence others and create a positive ripple effect in our communities. The act of being kind not only benefits others but also enriches our own lives, fostering a sense of connection and purpose.

Buddhism emphasizes the importance of compassion and loving-kindness (metta) towards all beings. This principle can guide our interactions, helping us treat others with empathy and respect. Simple acts of kindness, like smiling at a stranger, listening to a friend, or volunteering your time, can make a significant difference.

The great Buddhist teacher Nichiren Daishonin encouraged his followers over 700 years ago that lighting a lamp for another would also brighten their own way. In a sense, he's saying that kindness brings its own reward.

Volunteering at a food bank, tutoring students, or mentoring scouts, all of these are ways you can put kindness into action.

Modeling kindness starts with being kind to yourself. It can be hard to find compassion for ourselves, especially when facing the physical and emotional challenges of aging. We might also have internalized the criticism of others. And that tape might still be playing over and over in our heads.

I once co-led a personal growth seminar in which we talked about some of these old messages we carry around. When asked if anyone could identify what the source of these old self-criticisms might be, a middle-aged woman's hand shot up. "Oh yeah, I know exactly whose voice it is that I hear in my head. It's Sister Mary Margaret. In the 4th grade she told me that I'd never amount to anything."

Sister Mary Margaret is long gone. But the tape was still playing in this person's head.

Identify any old self-criticisms and let them go. If you need to, write them down on a piece of paper. Seal them in an envelope. Take it outside and light it on fire. Watch it go up in smoke and with it, all your old, unhelpful messages.

It's important to recognize your own worth and treat yourself with the same gentleness you would extend to those you love. This self-care is crucial for maintaining your mental and emotional well-being.

When we model kindness, we set an example for younger generations. Many people think of older folks as mean, cranky, and even nasty. We know that's not true, but we've probably seen some of our age group tribe lose their cool in cringey and embarrassing ways.

My mom does not suffer fools gladly. But I was very proud of her when she shared this story of how she changed her attitude towards a hapless salesperson at a department store.

Mom was shopping for some clothes and the sales clerk was scrolling through her phone. My mom wasn't finding what she wanted and her calls for help were being ignored. So, she started to get really steamed up. And just as she was about to lower the boom on the salesgirl with a string of profanity, she stopped. She thought about a conversation she and I had about kindness. She took a deep breath and asked herself, "What would a nice person do in this situation?"

My mom, a Buddha in training!

Just stopping to think about being more compassionate changed her whole attitude.

Even old dogs can learn new tricks.

Young people learn from our actions, seeing how to treat others with respect and compassion. In this way, our legacy of kindness can continue long after we are gone, impacting future generations and contributing to a more compassionate world.

To integrate kindness into your daily routine, consider performing one intentional act of kindness each day. It doesn't have to be grand or elaborate; even small gestures can have a profound impact. Over time, these acts will become second nature, and you'll find that kindness flows more easily and abundantly in your life.

Accept Grace

Accepting grace can be one of the most challenging, yet rewarding, aspects of aging. Grace is about finding peace and dignity in the process of growing older, embracing our experiences and changes with acceptance rather than resistance. This acceptance doesn't mean giving up or becoming passive; rather, it's about understanding and appreciating the natural course of life.

Buddhism teaches us about the impermanence of all things (Anicca).

Everything in life is transient, including our youth, health, and even our loved ones. By accepting this impermanence, we can find a deeper sense of peace and contentment. This acceptance allows us to let go of unnecessary suffering and to appreciate the present moment for what it is.

Grace also involves forgiving ourselves and others. Holding onto grudges and regrets can weigh heavily on our hearts, especially as we age. By practicing forgiveness, we release this burden and open ourselves to healing and peace. Remember, forgiving doesn't mean condoning hurtful actions; it means freeing ourselves from the pain they have caused.

Finding grace in aging has the extra benefit of recognizing and valuing the wisdom and experience we have accumulated over the years. Society often focuses on the negatives of aging, but there is much to celebrate as well. Our experiences have shaped us into who we are today, and there is great value in sharing our stories and insights with others.

Grace can come to us in unexpected ways. A prism of light that colors a window, the laughter of a child, the smell of incense in a church, or the haunting music of a street busker can trigger in us a sense of the divine, a timeless connection to all things, and a deep sense of calm.

For some, engaging in reflective practices such as meditation or prayer can help cultivate this connection and a sense of inner peace amidst the changes of aging.

Bringing It All Together

Integrating the three core values of seeking beauty, modeling kindness, and accepting grace into your daily life can transform your experience of growing older. They provide a framework for finding joy and meaning, regardless of the challenges you may face.

Remember, it's never too late to start. Each day is an opportunity to practice these values and to grow in your understanding and appreciation of life. By seeking beauty, you open your heart to the wonders of the world. By modeling kindness, you spread joy and compassion to those around you. And by accepting grace, you find peace and dignity in the natural flow of life.

Aging is an inevitable part of the human experience, but how we approach it can make all the difference.

By embracing these principles, we can navigate the journey of aging with a vibrant, progressive spirit.

This approach not only enriches our own lives but also leaves a lasting positive impact on those we encounter. Take a moment to reflect on these values and consider how you can incorporate them into your life.

Growing old doesn't have to be something we dread. With the right mindset and practices, it can be a time of profound growth, wisdom, and joy. Embrace these values and let them guide you towards a fulfilling and beautiful journey through the later years of life.

Remember, you aren't dead yet – so stop acting like it! Live vibrantly now and savor all that life has to give you.

Chapter 12
Afterword

Daisaku Ikeda wrote, "The last years of our life are the most important. If those last few years are happy ones, we have had a happy life. The victories and achievements up to that time are all illusory; the person who wins in the end is a victor in the truest sense of the word."

I hope you have found the tips in this book to be helpful. If so, please recommend it to a friend. I would also appreciate it if you left a positive review on Amazon.com or wherever you found this book. A good review helps others find this book.

The last tip I have to share with you is simple: live intentionally. If you make intentional choices about how you want to spend your time, energy, and resources, you will have a more fulfilling and purposeful life.

None of us know how long we will be alive. If we live everyday as if it is a precious gift, we can age gracefully and joyfully.

There is still work to do, flowers to plant, children to hug, stories to record, and music to dance to. Now is the time.

The third stage of our lives can be one fraught with pain, resentment, and regret. Or, it can be a golden era where we put the finishing touches on our lives bathed in the rays of a magnificent sunset.

The choice is yours.

I choose to live vibrantly each day.

If you want to share your thoughts or continue the conversation, you can reach me at info@modernwisdom.com

Also by Marc J. Sachnoff

You might also enjoy these titles by Marc and his colleagues -- all available on Amazon.com

The Gift – A Revolution In Networking Master

Your True Path: Discover Your True Path to a Life of Success and Fulfillment

The End of Self- Doubt: Build Lasting Confidence and Self-Esteem with The Inner Compass Method

About the author

Marc J. Sachnoff

Two-time Emmy-Nominated Television Producer, entrepreneur, author, and humanitarian, Marc Sachnoff is a sought-after advisor, negotiator, and intuitive business strategist. Marc has provided services to organizations as diverse as Coca Cola, Microsoft, Precor, Oki Golf and the Presidential Inaugural Committee and worked as a Director of Business Development in Microsoft's Xbox gaming division. In his 4 decades of Buddhist practice in the SGI-USA Buddhist Association, Marc has served in many volunteer leadership positions locally and nationally. Marc lives in Seattle with his wife, one rescue dog, and six pianos.

www.ingramcontent.com/pod-product-compliance
Lightning Source LLC
Chambersburg PA
CBHW061801070526
44586CB00023B/2668